Rev. Dr. Mark. D. & Kathy M. Brown, I.

Dynamic Muscular Breakthrough

Technology©

1000 PEOPLE Will Die Today From

Obesity Related Diseases!

This Generation's CHILDREN Are

Supposed To Die Before Their

PARENT'S

We Will Not Stand By & Let The

CHILDREN

DY-BUTT, ©Our New

DYBUTT Products Are

GOING to SAVE THIER LIVES!

# Dynamic Muscular Breakthrough Technology©

1000 PEOPLE Will Die Today From Obesity Related Diseases!

This Generation's CHILDREN Are Supposed To Die Before Their PARENT'S

We Will Not Stand By & Let All Of You DY-BUTT, ©

Our New DYBUTT© Products Are GOING to SAVE THEIR LIVES!

Rev. Dr. Mark. D. & Kathy M. Brown,I.

Published by MD& KM Brown, I. Publishing©

# Copyright© 2009 by Rev. Dr. Mark D. & Kathy M. Brown, I.

Rev. Dr. Mark. D. & Kathy M. Brown, I.

Dynamic Muscular Breakthrough Technology©

1000 PEOPLE Will Die Today From Obesity Related Diseases!

This Generation's CHILDREN Are Supposed To Die Before Their

PARENT'S

We Will Not Stand By & Let All Of You

DY-BUTT, ©

Our New DYBUTT Products Are

GOING to SAVE YOUR LIVES!

Unless otherwise indicated, Bible quotes are taken from The King James Version, copyright©
1997 by Word publishing, and the New American Standard Bible, copyrigh©1960 by
Harvest House Publishers. Definitions were obtained from the Merriam-Webster's online
dictionary and Bible. Kathleen Brown's material is from her upcoming book to be named later.
All data from the Center for Disease Control is from their website. All information from the
Web Geek is from their website. Trends in Obesity-Related Deaths and Cardiovascular Risk,
are from the Journal Watch website. The surgeon general information came from the US Department
Of Health and Human Services office of the Surgeon General website
About.com articles by Laura Dolson from the About.com website.

## Dynamic Muscular (DYBUTT) Breakthrough Technology

"My people are destroyed for lack of knowledge: because thou hast rejected knowledge, I will also reject thee, that thou shalt be no priest to me: seeing thou hast forgotten the law of thy GOD, I will also forget thy children." (Hosea 4:6 KJV).

# Sometimes the Things That You Think You Need the Most Are Already inside of You!

## You Just Need to CHALLENGE Yourself to Really Look Deep inside!

## Can you face the real YOU!

This book will show us how to harness the dynamic forces that have been lying dormant deep inside of our country's & OUR unified bodies for the last 35 years and is now ready to be awakened to a new level of physical fitness and health that has been long overdue. We are supposed to DY-BUTT we refuse to DY-BUTT WE ARE CHOSING TO LIVE. JOIN THE DY-BUTT MOVEMENT AND START LIVING NOW!!! Don't DYBUTT START DOING DYBUTT AND LIVE! DO DYBUTT AND LIVE NOW!

Mark & Kathy Brown, I. saw the reports, 1000 people are supposed to die from obesity related diseases every day. This is supposed to be the first generation that is going to die before their parents. That means that every hour 41 people would die from obesity related diseases! That means that every 90 seconds one person would die from obesity or fat related illnesses. That means that moms and dads would be burying sons and daughters! But there is a way out! But there is a way of escape! And we found it! Read on so you to can get out NOW! Read on so you can ESCAPE NOW!

## Dynamic Muscular (DYBUTT) Breakthrough Technology

Calling upon their over 50 years of combined fitness experience, their over 30 years of full potential development training and over 19 years of being in the Ministry, Mark and Kathy have developed a fitness program like no other. Because it is not just a workout program or a fitness program but it is a philosophy built upon not accepting any of the old if, and or but excuses for not being successful in whatever it is that you attempt including fitness and exercise.

Once one has had the Dynamic Muscular Breakthrough Technology© or DYBUTT© philosophy explained to them their life will never be the same!
One will have a new understanding and perspective on how to handle every problem and struggle that comes up in their lives!

This is the most efficient, the most effective, the newest, the greatest, the best, the most innovative, the freshest, and safest fitness experience that you will ever have! Start using the technology of the 21st century NOW! **GET INVOLVED WITH DYBUTT NOW AND START SAVING LIVES TODAY!**

## DYBUTT© IT IS GOING TO CHANGE YOUR LIFE!

## Dynamic Muscular (DYBUTT) Breakthrough Technology

Kathy and Mark Brown, I. have worked closely for many years at helping people reach their full potential and enhancing the quality of life of these individuals.

They have enhanced many people's lives with the radio programs that they hosted, the many speaking engagements that they have participated in and as former pastors of a church that they have founded.

It is Kathy and Mark's mission to eliminate this epidemic of obesity that is plaguing our nation as a whole and our youth in particular! They believe that with the right kind of education and training this can be done.

We have too many resources and too many smart, intelligent, hard working and dedicated people in our nation to allow such an easy foe to beat to overcome us, America.

We must start attacking this problem NOW! God bless America, and God bless you!

# Table Of Contents

## Acknowledgments

To my precious mother Ella Brown, who has gone on to be with the Lord, and my father Alonzo Brown.  There are not enough words to repay you for the examples that you set for my brothers and sister and myself of what it takes to be successful in life.

I want to thank you for letting me know that no matter what obstacles you face, no matter how daunting the adversary, no matter how much resistance you might encounter, you must never give up!

To help all of us understand that even though others may not appreciate what you are doing you cannot allow their opinion or their discouragement to define who you are or what you are doing!

I am extremely and eternally grateful for the opportunity to be part of your family and to call myself the son of Alonzo and Ella Brown.

To my dearly beloved and departed father Jake and my loving mother Fannie McNair, words cannot explain the depths of love or pride that I feel when I think of all the things that being a daughter has taught me and the other family members.

We are also grateful for the many sacrifices that you made for us because you both loved us so much.

## Dynamic Muscular (DYBUTT) Breakthrough Technology

I know that I speak for all of my brothers and sisters when I say that we are so very glad that we could bear and share your name. When I think of our family heritage and history and how so many have done well in life I can only think of one source that we all had in common and that was our tremendous family life. I will ever be grateful and proud to call myself your daughter, Kathy.

To my sisters and brothers Gladys, Carol, Joe, Ira, Dorothy, Jake, Belinda, Cynthia, & Robin; I will always be indebted to you all for the many things that we have shared as a family and experiences that we have gone through together.

You all have always been there for me to offer your support, concern and also your protection. Like mama used to always say *"if it doesn't kill you it will make you better"*

You guys are the reason that I am proud to be part of our family and I want to thank all of you from the bottom of my heart for all that you've done for me through the years and for all that we have shared as a family! I am so proud and glad to be your sister, love Kathy.

To my brothers Alonzo, James and Richard, and to my special sister Violet: I want to thank you all for looking out for your little baby brother. To this day I use a lot of what I learned from you to help me make it in life.

From the bottom of my heart and with everything that I have within me I want to express my heartfelt gratitude and my extreme pride for being able to say that I am your little brother.  Thank you, Mark

# <u>Dedication</u>

To our grandparents, mothers and fathers, our sisters and brothers, our children and grandchildren we want to thank you for your support and encouragement in this tremendous process!
To all of the political leaders, especially Senator Kirk Schuring, Congressman John Boccieri, Steven M. Meeks, Mayor William Healy thank you very much for your support!

To the local educators, principals Mr. Mark Black, Mr. Sandy Womack and Mr. Richard Brown thank you so very much for your vision, understanding & encouragement!
**Thank you, Sarge Robert Easley, Lets do this!**
**Thank you, Betty Smith, It is going to happen!**
**Thank you, Bill Luntz, my oldest student!**
**Thank you, Ray Strain for your inspiration!**
**We would most of all like to thank the school of hard knocks and criticism because you are the driving force that makes us wake up every day determined not to let 1000 DY-BUTT Live! Determined not to let the children DY-BUTT Live! WE WILL NOT GIVE UP UNTIL EVERYONE IS DOING DYBUTT & LIVING! DYBUTT IS GOING TO CHANGE THE WAY THE WORLD WORKS OUT! LET IT CHANGE YOUR LIFE TODAY!**

## Chapter1 How Many Are Dying?

In a Journal Watch article entitled Trends in Obesity-Related Deaths and Cardiovascular Risk, (Journal Watch Cardiology April 23, 2004) it was noted that that the Center for Disease Control researchers reported in 2004 that lack of exercise and a bad diet accounted for more than 400,000 US deaths in 2000. They have since corrected that figure to 365,000(JAMA 2005: 293:298).

In another study it was estimated that obesity accounted for 112,000 excess deaths every year in the US.

Whatever the actual number of deaths that can be attributed to poor diet and lack of exercise are; whether it's 112,000, 365,000, or 400,000 that is not just a number or statistic, but each number or statistic represents a person that has died needlessly.

Especially in this day and age of supposed better knowledge about obesity, fitness, health, healthy food choices, fitness gurus on every corner, healthy meal plans, fitness and food infomercials on every channel during all times of day and night, why are we still seeing so many people becoming obese and experiencing the tragic results of that obese lifestyle that can ultimately end in their deaths.

The US Department of Health and Human Services Office of the Surgeon General reported on the www.hhs.gov site that 61% of all U.S. adults were overweight in 1999. It was also reported that approximately 300,000 deaths each year in the United States might be attributed to obesity.

The report went on to reveal that 40% of all adults in the United States do not participate in any leisure time physical activity. Of that percentage, less than one third of them engaged in the recommended amount of at least 30 minutes of moderate to vigorous physical activity for most days.

In his recent addresses to the nation in March of 2009, our newly elected President, President Obama made the statemant that if our nation can get back to the obesity standards of the 1980s that we would be in good physical shape & eliminate some of the major health concerns we have.

It appears that almost everyone in the United States of America, from fitness and health gurus, the Center for Disease Control, doctors, the Surgeon General, and even the President of the United States himself is concerned about this rising trend known as the obesity epidemic!

Then if we couple that with the multiple millions and maybe even billions of dollars that we spend every year on fitness equipment, club memberships, exercise equipment, exercise DVDs, personal trainers, special diets, exercise clothing and the like. One has to wonder how can a nation that seems to be using so many resources and has brought to the attention of its population the need to eat correctly and to indulge in proper exercise, can be facing an obesity and fitness calamity!

It almost seems as if the more information we have and the more money and resources we allocate to this particular problem the more adults and children we have becoming obese and dying everyday!

Our children seem to be getting larger and larger, a recent Center for Disease Control study showed that 16% of all adolescents ages two to 19 were obese. It also showed that 31% of all adult males were obese and that 33% all women were obese.

It was also noted in this study that the health consequences of being obese were these:

- Coronary Heart Disease
- Type 2 Diabetes
- Cancer (endometrial, breast, and colon)
- Hypertension (high blood pressure)
- Dyslipidemia (high total cholesterol or high levels of triglycerides)
  Stroke
- Liver and Gallbladder Disease
- Sleep Apnea and Respiratory Problems
- Osteoarthritis (a degeneration of cartilage & its underlying bone within a joint.
- Gynecological Problems (abnormal menses, infertility)

Those are but a few of the health risks and diseases that come with being overweight. I'm sure that's there are many more that you are aware of just as I am but that's enough to let us understand about all the dangers that are inherent when one becomes obese or too fat!

It is not my hope to cause anyone any pain or suffering when I use the terms obese or fat. I do not have a dislike for nor do I feel anything but love and concern for all of my obese, overweight, or fat brothers and sisters. It is a problem that I encountered after I'd been in an automobile accident late in life.

God had to show me "but for his grace there go I". There is an old saying and I'm going to paraphrase it, *never judge a man until you walk in his shoes or moccasins for one day*. I would put quotation marks around it but I don't know who said it. But it's an extremely good saying because when I experienced what it was like to be overweight, obese, or fat I truly had a better understanding of the condition and also of the feelings that often come along with the condition.

I just wanted to make it clear to everyone that when we allow ourselves to get into this condition that there are many very detrimental things that can happen to us. I use the word allow here because that's exactly what most of us do, we permit this condition to occur. I know that's what I did and again that's what most of us do.

However, there is some new research from the Center for Disease Control that I would like to share with you about the role that genetics may play in one becoming obese. I was going to paste it here but it won't copy completely. You can go to their website at www.cdc.gov/ features/obesity.

To provide you with a summary of what the article says it is letting us know that the gene called the Thrifty Gene, prominent in the "Thrifty Genotype" Hypotheses, the same gene that helped our ancestors survive occasional famines are now being challenged by environments in which food is plentiful year round. The thrifty gene in theory may be preventing us from losing weight because it's storing or hoarding our fat like it would if we were living during a famine.

But and we say BUTT we're not buying that theory! We think that generally, if we read the article, they say identifying those factors that support this theory of obesity being based upon the genetic factors of fat hoarding has been difficult to prove. So at best I think we can give the theory a farfetched maybe, pending more research.

But that brings up the other exciting part of the research in the article, which used family history to reflect genetics susceptibility and environmental exposures shared by close relatives to prepare a family health history to identify people at high risk of obesity related disorders such as diabetes or cardiovascular diseases and some forms of cancers.

Since this group would be aware that they were at high risk for these type of disorders, they would be aware of the fact that they would need to be especially careful and avoid conditions and situations which would cause them to put on any extra weight. I am praying that they can do this so that they will not DY-BUTT LIVE.

# Chapter 2    Who Are You?

Butt it still comes back to knowing who you are doesn't it?  We can and I say we, because even though it was, for a relatively brief period of time, nevertheless I was overweight, obese, fat. And I am not criticizing, making fun of, belittling, browbeating, chastising or in any way condemning you because I am one of you. I feel your pain and I know you suffering brothers and sisters.

And I believe that everyone is a miracle of God and that God has taken great pains to make sure that everybody, no matter who you are, has been created to do something and be something special! When we think about the fact that he gave his only begotten son for us we can only conclude that he felt that we were something special.

We find in the words that he inspired in the Bible, that are recorded in Psalms 139:14 a very clear expression of whom God thinks we are, and what he thinks we are.  For it reads, *"I will praise thee for I am fearfully and wonderfully made marvelous are thy works and that my soul knoweth right well"*.  What this verse means is that all persons have been created by God to be awesome and outstanding!  The miracle of life is nothing short of being mind-boggling! Just to consider all of the different processes that go on inside of the human body and what it can do is mind-boggling, will blow your mind and is truly amazing.

All human beings truly are a medical marvel, the way we can move and adapt to many different circumstances and situations. We have the adroitness to be able to pick up a tiny piece of hair much smaller than a pinhead and the brute strength and force to be able to push a car that weighs a ton! We can dance on the tips of our toes as a dainty ballerina or slam-dunk on a 14-foot rim like a powerful basketball player!

We have the capacity to be able to run for miles as the great marathoners or extreme endurance athletes and we can swim in the water as a great Olympians. Our bodies have the ability to generate and withstand tremendous collisions such as those involved in football but also can avoid colliding with one another on the dance floor! One second we can accelerate and run at full speed but then just as quickly we can decelerate and come to a complete stop!

What is really amazing is not so much all the things that we can do but the relatively few things that we cannot do. We human beings & our bodies are AWESOME, AWE INSPIRING AND WONDERFULL! GO TO YOUR MIRROR RIGHT NOW AND TELL YOURSELF HOW GREAT YOU ARE! TELLYOURSELF HOW WONDERFULL YOU ARE! DON"T LET ANOTHER SECOND PASS, DO IT NOW!

If you notice the last part of Psalms 139: 14 it states and that my soul knoweth right well. In other words the Psalmists is explaining that he knows this deep down in his soul and he knows it totally or completely. You need to totally and completely know how special you and your fearfully and wonderfully made bodies are.

Even if you do not believe in God you still must admit that human beings and our bodies are great, wonderful, awesome, or as Michael Jackson used to say *" we're Bad, Bad really really BAD!"*

*And that's GOOD!* We just need to appreciate this fantastic and marvelous body that we have and we must begin to treat it as such.

I want us to think about something for me right now. I want us to think about the most valuable car that we have or about the most valuable car that we could have. Say this car is the most expensive Cadillac that we could buy. This car had cost us, after we had put all the accessories on it, $80,000. This was your dream car and it was beautiful from the ground up! This car was awesome, this car was clean, this car was nice, and this car was *BAAAD!*

You had cleaned your car up, polished it so good that it was shining in the sunshine like a beautiful brand-new diamond. When you looked at it you had to put on sunglasses because it was so bright! You had meticulously cleaned the interior and the carpets looked like they were as new as when you bought the car. The wood veneer had been polished and would make any piece of furniture in your house jealous because it looked so good.

The windows were so clean that you couldn't tell if they were rolled up or rolled down. You had

24

even made sure that the pushbuttons on the power windows and locks were shining like new money. The vehicle was immaculate and because you're taking your time to do such an outstanding job you were, to say the least, extremely proud of the job you had done and with the present appearance of your vehicle. It took you about four hours from start to finish, BUT you thought that it was worth your efforts.

It was a bright sunny day and on such days after you had detailed your car, you liked to take a 10-minute or so drive around your neighborhood just to do a little showing off because you knew, you knew that you and your car would be looking GOOOOOD!

Out of the corner of your eye you notice someone is coming toward you at a very brisk pace, it's your neighbor and he's been out running with his dog. He's been after you trying to get you to give him and his dog a ride in your beautiful, clean, immaculate & BAAAD vehicle.

But so far you've been avoiding him and his dog because you know that when they go out running he and the dog like to roll around in the field where the horses are. Sometimes your neighbor and his dog get horse waste on themselves when they do this!

Before you can get away, before you can get into your beautiful vehicle, your neighbor and his dog are right next to you. Your neighbor pops the question, when are you going to let me and spot take a ride with you in this beautiful, immaculate and bad vehicle? You can smell, I mean tell that they had been rolling in the field and were plenty dirty.

You think about the amount of effort that you put into detailing this beautiful vehicle. All the time you took cleaning the interior, the wood veneer, the carpet, the windows, even the little buttons on the power windows. As dirty as they are and smell you're thinking that you know what they're going to do to the interior of the car, heck they might even get the outside of the vehicle dirty! What nerve, who in their right mind would ask you for ride in your vehicle in that condition?

In your mind's eye you can see the word *"NEVER"* very clearly and it's going to be coming out of your mouth very soon! Right now, at this moment, you have to make a choice. You must decide whether you will permit your dirty neighbor and his dirty dog to have a ride in your beautiful, clean, and precious vehicle. You are now at a crossroads and you must decide if you feel that your vehicle and keeping it clean is more important than hurting your neighbor's feelings.

You have several choices that you can make. You can tell your neighbor that he needs to go clean himself and his dog up and then you will give them a ride. You can tell your neighbor that he needs to go and clean himself and his dog up, and that he can have a ride, but not his dog. You can tell your neighbor NEVER, that there is no way in the world, in this life, that he or his dog will ever get to ride in your beautiful, clean, immaculate and precious vehicle.

Now I know that all of you would do the politically correct thing, the neighborly thing, and forget about all the effort, the time and the care that you put into meticulously detailing your vehicle.

I know that all of you would say neighbor, even though I spent almost four hours detailing this vehicle making sure that it was in immaculate condition. I made this vehicle looks so good today that it looks better than it did when it came off of the showroom floor! But neighbor because you are so very special to me, my neighbor, I'm going to take you and you dog for a ride right now with me and you don't even have to worry about cleaning up at all!

So what if you and your dog get the carpet dirty, I'll just clean it again. So what if you and your dog get horse waste on my beautiful leather seats. I just have to work a little harder and scrub a little harder but I'll get it clean neighbor. Because you are my neighbor and I love you and your dog a lot. Now I bet that's exactly what you would do isn't it! Yeah, sure, right tell me another one. I don't know exactly what words would be used when discussing this issue with our neighbor.

BUT I am sure that we would CHOSE to do everything we could to keep him and his dog out of our precious, beautiful vehicle.

# Chapter 3 Choices: What a Powerful Word

We take so much care and pride in things like vehicles or homes or furniture and we would not blink an eye when it came to telling someone not to abuse our carpet or furniture. I wish I had a dime for every time I heard the words you'd better make sure you take your shoes off or wipe your feet off good before you come into my house! Or please put a coaster under your glass and thank you. Please don't smoke in my car because you're going to make it stank like cigarette smoke. Any of those sound familiar? I bet they do!

The reason why we do this is because we believe that these things are valuable, beautiful, important and precious. To the point that we choose to treat them with respect, dignity and as if they are valuable. And because of this choice that we make to value them, we will also demand that others treat them with respect, dignity and value. Furthermore if they don't respect these things we will even go as far as to ask them out of our vehicle, our house or our lives.

Choices, when we decide to make them and stick to them we can make a significant difference in the way that things are treated and most importantly the way that we are treated! We just have to understand that we must make the right choices to receive the right outcome that we are looking for in our lives.

Why do we choose to put so much importance on protecting and preserving a house, furniture, carpet, or a vehicle when we don't put the same kind of value on ourselves? We find out that it is not healthy for us to smoke and that smoking will cause us to have a laundry list of diseases, and yet we still have people who are smoking like crazy. But there is an underlying reason why people get hooked on cigarettes or the nicotine that is so prevalent in the cigarettes.

As is evident by the many different nicotine substitutes that are available now, it seems pretty clear that there is a very addictive side to smoking cigarettes. And I'm so glad that so many people are continuing to make the Choice of not smoking or to quit smoking if they already do because it is a very strong addiction to overcome.

They have realized that they are of more value than a house, a piece of carpet, a piece of furniture or a vehicle and they have Chosen to not put that smoke from the cigarette and it's related chemicals, in their great, beautiful, and precious bodies.

That's the same approach that all obese Americans must take in dealing with this "*Obesity Epidemic*", that we are facing right now. We must realize that just as the smoker has chosen to value himself more than he does that cigarette, the obese person must realize that they are more valuable and their health is more important and valuable than a piece of meat or that second helping or that desert!

But once we realize that then just like the smoker we may need to have something like the nicotine patches that would help us to cope with the symptoms of withdrawal as we fight this battle of the bulge. And I believe that I have found the secret weapon, the silver bullet, the thing that can be used when we are faced with the horrors of trying to wean ourselves from certain foods and limiting our food intake.

I'm going to clarify what that silver bullet, that secret weapon is, that if you will, food patch is. BUTT before I do I'd like to tell you a story.

We can seem to find so many different reasons why we cannot stop eating or why we cannot lose the weight and all of them come back to one thing and that's our choices! Even after I tell you about

31

the silver bullet that I have for obesity you will still have to make a choice of either following my advice or not following it. The choice will be yours.

This is one of the most powerful words in the world, choices. What we choose to do is going to determine what we become, how much of a success we are, what kind of a career or job we may have, the kind of person we become, who we will or will not marry, basically everything that we do in life will be governed by our choices. There are some random events that are out of our control BUTT; for the most part we are in control of our choices. Especially those that involve what we put in our mouths and where we take and what we do with our bodies!

Officers from the local police department, the detective unit, the bomb squad, SWAT, and the FBI surrounded the building. The suspect was moving about in the building and he had taken two hostages. The authorities began to move in closer and secured the perimeter of the building! The suspect had the hostages move in closer to him so that if he had to he would be able to use his deadly weapon upon them.

The hostages were now completely and totally under his control and they knew that they had to do whatever he said or he would use his dreaded weapon upon them. Any chances for them to escape were gone. Any hope of getting away had vanished and the only choice that they could make now was to choose to do exactly what the suspect ordered them to do. If they did anything else they knew that he would unleash the full force of his deadly weapon upon them!

All they could do now was pray for a miracle, for some type of holy intervention that would allow them to at least have a chance, have some hope because they knew that once he unleashed his weapon they would be through, finished, kaput, donya, it would be over for them!
This scene was playing itself out all over

America; people being taken hostage unwittingly by suspects just like this one, everywhere in America.

Most of the time the suspect or his kind would go in undetected and reek havoc on the unsuspecting victims, but lately, because they have been exposed on food labels everywhere, the authorities were starting to ferret them out. Consumers were also starting to become more educated and aware of their dirty tricks and also the areas that they frequented and hung out. More and more people were resisting them and exposing them for the vicious killers that they were!

Sharpshooters were now in position and had already been given the green light to shoot; they were just waiting for a clear shot to take the suspect out. For some strange reason the suspect turn his head just right for the two victims to move aside just enough for the sharpshooter to get the opening that he was waiting for as he slowly squeezed the trigger the bullet struck the suspect right between the eyes and he dropped to the floor motionless, the life quickly seeping out of him. The hostages quickly moved away from his lifeless body and ran into the arms of their loved ones. What a close call, we thought you were a goner said one of the loved ones. I'm so glad that our prayers were answered and you made it.

Why was everyone so relieved that the hostages had made it out okay and that the suspect did not have a chance to unleash his deadly weapon? What were they all so afraid of? Maybe the suspect's name will give us a clue. He's goes by many aliases, one is simple sugar, but most people know him by the ingredients, the weapon he injects into them known as FRUCTOSE! Why are all those who know about it so afraid of it and why is it so deadly? Let me tell you why!

In an article by Laura Dolson on About.com which had been reviewed by their Medical Review Board it stated, "Fructose, is a monosaccharide, which the body can use for energy, because it does not
cause blood sugar to rise tremendously, has a low glycemic index. It was once thought that fructose was a good substitute for sucrose (table sugar). However, the American Diabetes Association and nutritional experts have changed their minds about this.

A small amount of fructose, such as is found in most vegetables and fruits is not a bad thing. In fact, there is evidence that a little bit may help our body process glucose properly. However, consuming too much fructose at once seems to overwhelm the body's capacity to process it. The diets of our ancestors contained only very small amounts of fructose. These days, estimates are that about 10% of the modern diet comes from fructose.

What happens if we consume too much fructose? Most of the carbohydrates we eat are made up of chains of glucose. When glucose enters the bloodstream, the body releases insulin to help regulate it. Fructose, on the other hand, is processed in the liver. To greatly simplify the situation: When too much fructose enters the liver, the liver can't process it all fast enough for the body to use as sugar.

Instead, it starts MAKING FAT, you heard me right, it starts MAKING FAT from the fructose and sending it off into the bloodstream as triglycerides. This is the form that most fat is stored in the body". "Body fat is almost entirely made up of triglycerides, and fats are mostly transported in this form as well. Too many triglycerides in the blood and we have a great risk for heart disease. But let's get back to our old friend fructose.

"Why is this bad for us? As mentioned before high triglycerides are a risk factor for heart disease. The fructose ends up circumventing the normal appetite signaling system, so appetite-regulating hormones are not triggered and we are left feeling unsatisfied. This is probably at least part of the reason why excess fructose consumption is associated with weight gain.

There is also growing evidence that excess fructose consumption may facilitate insulin resistance, and eventually type 2 diabetes. However, some of this effect may be from chemicals in soda which reacts with high fructose corn syrup". Now we can see why the suspect had to be shot and why his victims felt so blessed to have escaped and remain alive.

**So the more of this stuff we eat the more of this stuff we want and we don't get the feeling that we are full or satisfied! So we just keep on eating more! WOW that's amazing!**
But there's more bad news and isn't that always the case! "What are the major sources of fructose? Fruit and vegetables have relatively small, normal amounts of fructose that our bodies

can handle quite well. The problem comes with the added sugars in the modern diet, the volume of which has grown rapidly in recent decades.

The blame has often been pinned to high fructose corn syrup (HFCS), which is made up of 55% fructose and 45% glucose. However, sucrose is the half fructose and half glucose. So, HFCS actually doesn't have a whole lot more fructose than a regular sugar, gram for gram. So what is the problem?

Why is this such a dangerous product? Don't we all like sweet things to eat? This is the major problem to this particular food item.
Today, almost all our foods have sugar added to them in some form, which almost always includes a lot of fructose. Honey has about to same fructose/glucose ratio as high fructose corn syrup. Fruit juice concentrates, sometimes used as healthy sweeteners usually have quite a lot of fructose and never mind that the processing of these concentrates strips away most of their nutritional value.

This is a product that is put into just about everything! And because of this we end up consuming small amounts of it's in many of our different products & the small amounts add up to a very large amount of the product when totaled together. Also remember that when we consume this product we do not feel as if we are satisfied or full and we want to eat more of the product. And because of this food companies find more products to put it in so that we become more deeply addicted to the product. Stay away from fructose, your choice.

Chapter 4   The Food Patch:  FRUITS & VEGTABLES

Well I told you earlier that I was going to tell you about the silver bullet, the secret weapon, *"the food patch"*. As noted in the previous article, fruits and vegetables in their normal state have the natural sweeteners in them that we crave. These natural sweeteners will allow our sweet cravings to feel satisfied and also provide us with the energy that we need to carry on with our everyday activities.

There are so many diets and really all a diet is supposed to be is the normal amount of food it takes for us to perform our daily activities without having a surplus of calories or a deficit of calories at the end of our day. So when we think of or discuss a diet lets use that definition as the one that we focus on. Now we can all be on the same page and speak in the same terms.

Most dietitians would tell us that a healthy protein, carbohydrate and fat ratio is necessary to have a balanced diet and one that will provide the right amount of nutrition and energy that your body needs to function throughout the day. The normal ratio is 40% carbohydrates, 30% protein and 30% fats give or take a couple of percentage points. The problem arises whenever we try to

The problem arises whenever we try to live without some of these components. One of the best examples of this healthy ratio that I've found is located at wise Geek.com & I'd like to share it with you now:

Casual dining and fast food portions have worked with various fad diets to distort our understanding of what we should eat and in what portion sizes. There can be dangerous consequences from radically reducing or increasing our carb, protein, fat ratio over an extended period of time. Still, many experts focused on their diets focus on proper carb, protein, ratio.

Experts disagree on what the proper ratio is, but most agree it is 40 to 45%, carbohydrates, 20 to 30% protein and 30 to 35% fat each day. Each macronutrient is important so let's look at why. Carbs, short for carbohydrates, are a ready and easy supply of energy since they break down quickly. Most carbs will digest completely in about two hours. With that in mind, we should eat carbs that are high in fiber to slow the rush of sugar to the blood stream. Simple carbs, like low and no fat chips, cookies, and snacks are usually high in calories but low in nutrients like fiber. If eaten in excess, simple carbs will be stored as fat in the body. 41

This is where carbs get their bad reputation. carbs supply much-needed energy to the heart, brain and kidneys that is why they've played a prominent role in the healthy carb, protein, fat ratio. A severe lack of carbs will cause our bodies to take additional measures to get the energy it needs. Our bodies will attempt to remove the carbs from our muscles, causing muscle loss.

Protein should be eaten in portions about the size of a deck of cards. Three to four of these portions would provide 60 to 80 g. (2.1- 2.8 ounces) of the protein needed each day. If you are trying to build muscle it is a good idea to add a few more grams of protein each day to promote muscle growth. Children should also take in a little more protein.

Fats break down into the good, the bad and the ugly. The really horrible fats are transfats that should be avoided entirely. They promote an increase in low-density lipoprotein (LDL) cholesterol (the bad kind) and reduce high-density lipoprotein (HDL) cholesterol (the good kind). When looking to add fats to your diet be on the look out for those ingredients. Don't just rely on a label that says no trans-fat because foods with half a gram (0.02 ounce) of trans-fats or less are labeled as trans-fat free. Trans-fats include

42

anything that is hydrogenated or partially hydrogenated. Saturated fats are not as heart healthy as mono-unsaturated or polyunsaturated fats, but they are important and as much as 10% of our fat intake can come from saturated fats. You'll find that a lot of animal fats, including fat from dairy products, are saturated fats.

Finally, there's the good. Extra virgin olive oil is good for our hearts in moderation. Most nuts, canola, grape seed, and avocado oils are also good sources of fat. The usual rule of thumb for fats is you don't get a lot of them, so make them count. Whenever we examine what we should be eating we should be looking for a healthy carb protein fat ratio.

Our plates should be about one half healthy carbs such as a vegetable or salad, a one fourth lean protein like chicken, and finally one fourth should be a starchy food like bread, potatoes, or brown rice.

Another recommendation is to simply divide our plates into 3 equal parts. Fill with 1/3$^{rd}$ the plate with a protein source no bigger then the palm of your hand. Fill the other 2/3rds with vegetables & fruits. Eats some heart healthy nuts, extra virgin olive oil or some other heart healthy fat.

As we can see this is a tremendous article on not only describing why we need this ratio of carbs, protein and fat, but also what these different components of a balanced diet do for our bodies. And would you have guessed that we needed to have so much healthy fat in our daily diets to keep our hearts healthy? Or what about the amount of the portion of the protein that we need daily!

And then to consider the portion size, which is about the size of a deck of cards or the palm of your hand. Would you have ever thought that we need about the same percentage of fat as protein?

But now back to the super food, the silver bullet, *"The Food Patch"*. And I know you know what it is don't you. The Almighty Carbohydrate in its <u>Pure Unaltered Original State or Form</u>. Just as a smoker who is trying to quit smoking may occasionally have to have some additional help, and may not be able to go cold turkey, while trying to quit smoking. A food addict may occasionally need some help as well. This is our food addict's version of *"The Patch"*.

Everyone that has ever struggled with trying to lose any weight at all knows that there comes a point, almost every day that we get the urge to have a certain food. We call this urge a *"Craving"*. **No matter how stronged willed one maybe, if you're trying to lose weight one will be confronted with this great adversary, the craving!**

One may be tall, one may be short, one may be smart, one may feel as if they are not smart. One may be an executive, a laborer or any other kind of person, but if you're ever trying to change your eating habits and your daily diet for the better, you are going to experience a craving! And that craving will hit us like a ton of bricks.

Why is this happening? Because we are going through a withdrawal process which is not much unlike a heroin addict, or a crack addict, or an alcoholic or any other addicted person. So we may need to have a little help to ease the pain of this particular withdrawal process. And I know it may be hard to face the facts that we have an addiction as a nation, BUTT WE ARE ADDICTED TO FOOD!

# <u>Let me say that again, AMERICA, WE ARE ADDICTED TO FOOD AND</u>

45

# IF WE DON'T GET HELP SOON WE ARE GOING TO DIE!

America, we now have a channel that is dedicated to nothing but food. We can find almost any kind of food and how to prepare it on this channel. We have made those who are preparing this food on this channel stars and celebrities. If we were to think about food as an addicting substance, which it is. And the people who prepare that food as the pushers or drug dealers of that food, which they are. It's as if America, we have put the pushers or dealers on the air, are learning on a televised broadcast, from the pushers how to make the drug then have made the pushers stars and celebrities for showing us how to make the drug!

But that's not all American; we are also setting up distribution networks for this food drug by having elaborate dinner parties, lunches, brunches, barbecues and cookouts. And then we get instructions from them on how to increase our customer base in the form of these reports they let us buy called recipes & cookbooks! Oh yeah America they also write books on how to make more of this food drug & you get to buy those also! Aren't we the lucky ones?

And to add injury on to insult the same individuals open up elaborate facilities that they use to distribute more of their product. At these facilities they will personally make appearances and on occasion manufacture the product for you.

It costs a great deal of money to get the product from these facilities and there is always a great demand for the product because they always have big lines outside these facilities.
These facilities are known by the codename "restaurants".

My mother, God rest her soul, used to have a saying that she would say when I was young and I was eating too much. America, maybe some of you have heard it. She would say, "BOY WHAT ARE YOU TRYING TO DO? EAT YOURSELF TO DEATH?"

# <u>AMERICA, WHAT ARE WE TRYING TO DO? EAT OURSELVES TO DEATH?</u>

America, I asked some people about 30, when they found that they were the most susceptible to craving and they said while they were watching television. Think about that for a minute, ok, times up.

But the good news America is that we are now aware of the problem aren't we!  And now that we are aware of the problem we can start on the process of recovery from this addiction that we have.  So what should the first step of our recovery plan involve?  What will we start on first?

The first thing that most people who go into drug rehabilitation is told is to make sure that they changed their surroundings or their environment. They are told not to go around the same old friends, the same old hangouts, or do not watch the same type of materials that they used to watch. In other words America, we have to stop going to restaurants as much.  We have to stop watching food programs.  We have to stop watching so much television. Leave food magazines alone.

We have to stop buying food books and recipe books.  When we know that we are going to be in an environment where there is going to be a lot of food, we must avoid those areas where the food is located and spend our time in other areas.

48

America, we must also make sure that we avoid those areas where the smell of the food is very strong! Because as we all know we have all given in to many food temptations and cravings because the food smelled ***SOOOO GOOOOD!*** **DON'T LET YOUR NOSE BLOW YOUR GOALS!**

The next thing we must do America, is to start eating the right foods and in the right ratio as I outlined in the previous pages. Do not try any of those fad diets or drugs to help you lose weight quickly. We did not get in this condition overnight we will not get out of it overnight! A safe weight loss is about 2 to 4 pounds per week of fat. About a half a pound a day BUTT if we don't lose that, then do the best that we can!

America, we must not look at this as a quick fix or a temporary situation. Because I know there are many of us who get a goal in mind. We eat unhealthy or starve ourselves and do without food for longer then we normally should, and can maintain, we reach that goal and then we start to eat like crazy & gain all the weight back & then some! America if we don't do so good one day that's ok, just start over tomorrow, don't give up.

We all know the famous celebrity who has been on a roller coaster ride with weight issues and fitness issues for most of her career on television. She loses weights in vast amounts and chunks and then she gains weights in vast amounts and chunks. Our hearts goes out to her and we wish that we could sit down with her for about a week and talk with her about real health, real fitness and a lifelong process of change, especially in the areas of her fitness and her health.

One of the many things that we would share with her would be how the body becomes fat. When we eat a meal we turn everything we eat into glucose & it enters our bloodstream. This glucose is the primary source of energy for our bodies & our brains. Our pancreas releases insulin to go get this glucose and put it into our cells as energy.

Think of the insulin as a patrolman or a policeman on a motorcycle. This patrolman goes out and gets the glucose and attempts to put it into our cells as energy. If the cell is not full of glucose and needs the glucose it will open up a little cell door and let the patrolman put in the glucose. Our bodies use this glucose energy as fuel to do our daily tasks and functions through the day. However, if the cell is already full of glucose then the cell door will not open and the patrolman will not be able to put the glucose into the cell. Now the patrolman has a problem because he knows how valuable the glucose, or energy is to the body and that he cannot just throw this valuable energy source away, the patrolman must find someplace to store this energy. So what does the patrolman do?

America, you already guessed didn't you? The patrolman takes the glucose or energy source and he stores it on our hips doesn't he. BOY, DOES HE STORE IT ON OUR HIPS! Okay America, we eat another meal, it's converted to glucose and now more glucose, energy, is released into our bloodstream. Here comes the patrolman and he gets the glucose & tries to put it into the cell, BUTT the cell is full and the cell door will not open so what does the patrolman do? He must find a place to store it so he goes back to our hips and tries to store it there.

The hip area is full so the policeman must find another place to store this glucose energy, so now what does he do? He starts to store it on our abdomen, when that area fills up he will start to store it on other areas such as our thighs, under our chin, under our arms, on our back and then just about any and everywhere that he can. The patrolman will do this until he runs out of new places to store the energy & then what will happen.

YOU GET SO BIG UNTIL YOU EXPLODE & GO BOOM!  I'M just kidding, I'm just kidding, BUTT seriously, what really happens is that the patrolman starts to put the glucose energy on top of the areas that he has already put it on and so we get bigger and bigger or fatter & fatter. Now we have so much glucose energy and fat floating around in our system that we either get heart disease, sugar diabetes, have a stroke, get cancer, have an aneurysm or some other obesity related disease and end up dying because of that disease! What can we do to get rid of this horrible obesity epidemic curse, America?

Chapter 5    Reversing The Food Curse

What did we learn from the previous pages and how can they benefit us?  I don't know about you but I think I learned that the policeman is the one sticking too much fat on our bodies and that he must be eliminated!  He must be destroyed, let's go get the policeman!
Does anybody out there have an extra gun and a motorcycle?  If you do let me have it because I'm going to get that patrolman right now!

The most important thing to learn from the previous pages is that fat is nothing more than stored energy.  It is very important for us to not think of ourselves as being fat, BUTT let us think of ourselves now as being full of energy. As a matter of fact, some of us might say we have a surplus of energy. Some of us might say that we have an over abundance of energy and that we don't need to accumulate any more energy for a lifetime! No I'm just playing with you America I'm just kidding! I know that this is a very serious problem and I feel your pain and I'm here to help you with your over abundance of energy problem. Let's not call it fat for now; but let's call it

"Abundant Energy".

When we think of it in that manner maybe we can see and understand the problem a bit more clearly.

We must realize that we have to limit the amount of food energy that we consume so that when it is taken into our system and converted into glucose energy we only have what we need to function for the day. If we have a lot of abundant energy to get rid of and if we use the approach of only taking in the amount of energy that we need to function during the day, we will basically stay the same and our weight will not change. If our quest is to lose weight then this is not a very good approach. But what can we do to jumpstart our weight loss program through eating and get rid of this abundant energy?

Well I'm glad you asked that question because I have the answer for you and I'm excited about it. Just as the insulin patrolman was responsible for getting the glucose and putting it where it would best be utilized, there is also another fat friendly hormone to aid us in the battle of the bulge. Its name is glucagon and it is great!

Let's evaluate the problem America so that we can come up with a viable solution that is going to help us reverse this curse and prevent us from dying from this epidemic of obesity.

Before we talk about glucagon I want to tell you about another part of this process. Our bodies have the ability to store up to 400 g of glucose; the liver holds 100 g and the muscles hold up to 300 g. or about 1600 calories. If we burn up or consume these 400 g of glucose the insulin patrolman will put the glucose in the liver and the muscles to be used as fuel or energy for our bodies to function properly. However, if we do not burn up this 400 g of glucose in our cells, our liver and muscles will not open and the insulin policeman will store the glucose as fat. And America, we do not want that, no more Fat!

So what do we have to do America to stop this fat storage from happening? First we have to stop that insulin policeman from being released and how do we do that? Well since he is released when we increase the levels of carbohydrates in our system, then we need to decrease the level of carbohydrates that we consume!

High-fives all around and great big applause for
Mark and Kathy right! We did it and we are so
happy, congratulations, great job, celebration!

Butt there is only one problem; we need 40%
carbohydrates to have a balanced ratio in our diet!
If we mess that up then our bodies will
compensate by Robbing nutrients it needs from
other parts of our bodies. So we can stop all the
celebrating and go back to the drawing board
because, excuse my French but *"WE AIN'T
DONE YET HUN!"*
We need to eat carbohydrates but we need to
decrease the effects of the carbohydrates so that
the insulin police will not come out and get us.
We also need to find some way to burn up our
bodies' stored energy.
This is a fine mess you've got us in Mark, what
you *gonna* do now?

Think, think, think, think, not all carbohydrates
cause the insulin police to come out and get us
and store them somewhere as fats. As a matter of
fact those carbohydrates with a low glycemic
index number of 69 or less will keep the insulin
police at bay. What are these types of foods, most
fruits and vegetables but get a glycemic index
table to be sure.
Next we need to find a way to burn up all that

stored energy.

This is where our hero, our star GLUCAGON comes in! It is a fat burning hormone that is secreted by the pancreas to rise blood glucose levels by liberating stored glucose from the liver And Muscle Tissues! It also acts to stimulate the breakdown of fat energy and helps to stop The Storage Of Fat! But there is a catch Kathy, well Mark, when you're a woman dealing with a man, there always is! Are right what is it! Kathy, along with the low glycemic carbs we must exercise & it must be exercise that puts a load on our heart & lungs. Vigorous exercise!
To release our hero Glucagon, we must EXERCISE VIGOROUSLY!

What do you mean by vigorous exercise Mark? Do I have to go out and run a marathon or a triathlon or something? Do I have to go out and play a couple of matches of tennis or racquetball or squash or basketball? Do I have to swim for an hour or so? Can I just go out and take a nice leisurely walk or even a brisk walk, how about that Mark? What about some high impact aerobics like the classes down at the club? You know I have a slight knee problem and foot problem so I can't do a lot of jumping and running.

Well Kathy, most of those exercises that you have listed are very good and vigorous but they will definitely aggravate your knee and foot problems. The problem with walking even briskly is that the average person only walks fast enough to burn up 100 calories per mile; there are 3500 calories in a pound. At that rate a person would have to walk 35 miles to burn up one pound! That's a lot of walking! What type of exercise is one vigorous enough to burn fat and tone muscle, but gentle to the joints, ligaments, tendons, and cartilage?

Chapter 6   America's Favorite Workout!

Hello America, Mark and I are trying to find a fitness and workout program that would help us to be able to work out at a vigorous enough level that will enable us to release glucagon and start our internal fat burning process. It must be a workout or fitness experience that is also safe on our joints but tough and vigorous on our muscles. Do you know of anything like that America?

Well Kathy how did America responding to our question about the fitness program?  Actually Mark, we didn't get a very good response because most of the people, about 66% of them said they don't do any exercise at all! No wonder about 66% of the American population is overweight! I was very disappointed in them and the rest that responded were doing a little walking & some jogging. Very few were doing a muscle toning/building component.  They don't seem to understand that we need both to have a well-rounded fitness program.  Most people are just basically doing some form of an aerobic activity alone.

Well, Kathy, while we're in the mood for doing an intervention for food we might as well add the other addiction that we have in America and that is this:

# AMERICA, WE ARE ADDICTED TO WATCHING EVENTS AND JUST SITTING AROUND!

# WE JUST LOVE TO HANG OUT, CHILL OUT, AND VEG OUT, ZONE OUT, COOL OUT, TAKE OUT   TEXT OUT AND JUST DROP OUT!

# But If We Don't Get Help We Will Die Out!

We hate to be so blunt about this situation Butt when we are faced with an epidemic of the likes that we are facing; it is time for drastic action! It is time to take off the kid gloves, put on the boxing gloves and slap America in the face with the realities. We are a nation of great people, which was built upon the backs, the blood, sweat, and yes the tears of hard work and even harder workers.

A tough nation that was forged in the Civil War and protest, fighting for nothing more than a chance to be treated fairly and equally. Never looking for a handout but always looking for a fair shake and willing to work hard once we were given the opportunity so as to show our appreciation for that chance. We've been through depression, wars, terrorist attacks, economic downturns and many other things, but none of those things could stop or destroy us, We Are Still Here.

We were a nation that always enjoyed competition in all arenas of life and we always competed to win and were leaders in business, in commerce, in innovation, in academics and especially in athletics.

America's athletes were known all over the world for being ranked among the best in every sport. Who can forget how Jesse Owens represented the superiority of the American athlete during the Berlin games, and gave Adolph Hitler and in your face with his outstanding performance. Truly American physical fitness and prowess was on display for the whole world to see, appreciate and marvel at that day! Truly, every American had to be proud to be an American that day!

BUTT somehow we have lost our way; we have seemed to have forgotten who we are and now we are just a shell of our former selves. We loved to compete in person, BUTT now we live vicariously through the athletes that we watch perform on television & in arenas or the ones we become while we are playing the video games.

We play all of these games in a world of virtual-reality, taking on the form of different powerful looking game figures. The men and women in these video games look like superhuman beings. They all look like bodybuilders with their huge muscles and slim waistlines!

Those games which feature these kinds of characters seem to be the most popular, so it would seem that if we could, we Americans would like to look like that or as close to it as were legally possible.

By that I mean without drugs or artificial means BUTT by the good old American way. Through good old American perseverance, hard work, dedication & know how!

America, let us tell you why it's so important to have a fitness program that involves both a cardiovascular and a muscle toning and building component. First of all we need to look at the cardiovascular component of a good fitness program. The reason why we need to have a good cardiovascular component to our fitness program America is because we need to have an exercise experience that will raise our heart rate and increased blood circulation throughout the body.

Cardiovascular exercise is also good for burning off access fat and helping us to maintain a consistent weight. Cardiovascular exercise improves our heart health. Our heart is a muscle just like any other; in order for it to become strong we must work it. If we fail to work it it will become weak and over time become susceptible to a variety of negative health effects. When our hearts are made to pump at a faster rate we will be able to get into shape and maintain that conditioning. The more we work our hearts the stronger they will become and the healthier we will become. Training our heart improves every aspect of our fitness.

Our hearts will become more efficient at moving oxygen and fuel to our muscles to maintain a higher level of performance. The muscles known as our skeletal muscles also become more efficient at removing oxygen from the bloodstream with continued consistent exercise, our cardiovascular system progressively gets better.

Another benefit of cardiovascular or aerobic training is that it will increase our metabolism, or the way our bodies manage and burn our calorie on a daily basis. The more intense the workout the more our metabolism will be affected by this workout. This will allow us to burn up our calories quicker and more efficiently. But cardiovascular exercise also improves our hormonal profile. It releases hormones that make us feel good and helps regulate symptoms associated with depression, anxiety and fatigue. It also helps to suppress our appetite and generally improves our outlook on life. Cardiovascular exercise is one of the greatest stress relievers that is known to man.

Cardio also improves our ability to recover from a strenuous lifting session or other type of hard work. Some athletes even use a session of cardio to make sure all their parts are working right and that they don't have any hidden injuries or trauma from a previous physical exertion. Cardio can also be very beneficial in delaying the onset of muscle stiffness or soreness associated with the completion of many physical contests. Cardio is also used as a warm-up before many physical contests.

Cardiovascular Exercise is also very good for managing and regulating different types of diseases such as diabetes. Cardiovascular exercise does this by increasing our muscles ability to utilize glucose. Regular exercise helps us better control our blood sugars. They do not seem to be as many blood sugar swings among those who have regular cardiovascular exercise sessions.

As you can see cardiovascular exercise is very important for helping us to be able to reach our fitness goals. It also is beneficial for us to activate the hormone Glucagon that will help us to be able to burn up fat. That is the main culprit that everyone wants to get rid! Fat! It is public enemy number one! Why is fat so hated and why is it so despised? If you have a moment I'd like to tell you about fat!

The two main areas for fat deposits are under the skin, subcutaneous fat or deep in the abdomen, surrounding organs such as the liver, kidneys, pancreas and small intestines. This type is known as visceral fat. Visceral fat is killer fat because it has direct access to liver, which turns it into cholesterol.

Visceral fat is also an active organ. It releases chemicals that cause inflammation in the arteries. Inflamed arteries become clogged arteries that increased the risk of heart disease, stroke, aneurysms, and high blood pressure.

Belly fat is dangerous because visceral fat causes it. Our cells are likely to be resistant to insulin, which put us at high risk for diabetes, heart attacks and premature deaths. Storing fat in our belly causes us to store excess fat in the liver, which interferes with the livers function to remove insulin from our bloodstream after it has done its job of driving the blood sugar into a cells or storing it as fat. If we become insulin resistant we can develop diabetes that can lead to a life of taking shots, popping pills, blindness, kidney failure, heart disease, high blood pressure, nerve damage, limb amputation and even death.

It is very important that we keep our waistlines as slim and fat free as possible to help us stop the risk associated with visceral or belly fat.

It is also imperative that we must encourage our youth to stay as fat free as possible so that we will be able to help them avoid the number one pitfall of most young children who are obese and that is becoming obese adults. Statistics have shown that obese children tend to become obese adults.

The Center For Disease Control has said that the life expectancy of this generation is shorter than that of their parents. This is the first time that that is supposed to occur. Diseases and illnesses that normally have been showing up in much older individuals are now commonly being diagnosed in our nation's children! Our youth are in the worst shape in our history and it seems as if there is no relief in sight.

They seem to be unmotivated by their physical education experiences in our schools and it seems as if the teachers are at their wits end as to what to do to motivate them. We must make it our mission to help them come to the realization that fitness needs to become a lifetime pursuit. We believe that if we start our children off on the right foot that it won't be long before they will develop the belief that fitness is just another part of their life, just like brushing their teeth. They will also feel that is important to do this for the rest of their lives. But why does it seem that our youth are so preoccupied with watching things like sports & not participating in them? Why is it that they're more inclined to sit back and observe rather than get out and do?

Why do we as a nation of doers, America, a nation that forged its way through many difficult frontiers and wildernesses with nothing but primitive tools and will power. Now seems content to sit around and watch, as life seems to be passing it by. Well, we have a very general theory and hypothesis as to why this is the case, America. This will probably be a subject of future study, discussion and even a very serious and in-depth study but for now it is just our theory, our hypothesis, our belief.

Chapter 7     Couch Potatoes:  Made In America

Have you ever watched a young child, America as he or she was beginning to discover how to crawl, stand, walk, & then finally run! Did you notice how they were so full of determination as they progressed through each step?  As they were learning to crawl they would go faster & faster building up their confidence as well as their little muscles and stamina. And with each new increase in their speed they seem to have experienced such great unadulterated joy and happiness.

It seemed as if they had discovered the greatest toy in the world, and they were determined to have as much fun with it as they possibly could. And you know what that toy was America?  It was their discovery of their ability to be able to manipulates, motivate and most of all to move their bodies in the direction that they wanted to. Answers.com defines locomotion as *1.  A self-propelled vehicle, usually electric or diesel powered, for pulling or pushing freight or passenger cars on a railroad track. 2. A driving or pulling force; an impetus: that player serves as a locomotive for our team!*

69

They seem to have learned, America that one of the greatest joys in the world that one can experience is the joy of movement in all of its various forms! It doesn't matter if a young child is crawling as babies do, or if it is running as some of our most exciting and graceful professional athletes do, just the sheer exhilaration one gets from moving our bodies is often times a truly breathtaking & enjoyable experience for its participants!

As a child begins to grow and gains more control of its body and it becomes able to turn from side to side and maneuver around tables and chairs. The child seems to be so content, happy but most of all excited and engaged in just the sheer pleasure and exhilaration that it receives from just moving! The child has no toy, telephone, computer, ipod, or any other game and the child is still completely engaged in what it is doing. The only thing that is engaging the child is ITSELF America, and that seems to be doing a very complete and thorough job!

As a child grows older America, now it has gone from the point of being able to crawl and now it can walk! The child can walk around the chairs, tables, coffee tables, end tables, TV table, bookshelves and all kinds of different objects. But the child not only grows in its abilities to be able to control his body, But the child's curiosity grows also.

When that happens the child now naturally starts to want to pick up objects and items and more and more and more objects and items! At this point it is common to hear the child's mother make statements such as, *"that little thing it just seems to get into everything."* Next thing you know America, the child wants to pick up some of these items from off the different tables. But there's a little problem, the child doesn't have quite the control over its fingers and hands, (or very good fine motor function).

Now the child wants to pick up some of these items and bring them to us and when it does we smile and to the child that is a sign of our approval and affection. The child, wanting to get more of our approval and affection decides to bring us more items and then it decides to bring us one of mommy's real little pretty, delicate and dainty and verrrrrrryy expensive items. But something happens to the item on the way to its destination, us.

The child breaks the item while it was on the way to bringing it to us, and we're not upset at the child because it was trying to please us, BUTT, and this is where our theory comes in, now we feel as if we must do something to prevent the child from getting into more mischief!

The first thing we do is pick the child up in an attempt to try to control where it can go & the things that it can get into. No more moving around freely and without a chaperone. We make a statement such as; you're going to stay up here with me so you can stop moving around so much and getting into trouble.

What we really have done is two things. Number one we have picked the child up & stopped it from moving around. Number two we have put in the child's mind that they need to stop moving around so much and getting into trouble, they now may associate moving around with trouble.

We then go out and buy little "**Playpens**" and used them as little **Kiddie jails** to make sure that the child doesn't move around so much & stays out of trouble. We have successfully put the child and its ability to move around on locked down! Just as the child was beginning to enjoy the great fun that one can get out of being able to manipulate and maneuver this fantastic piece of equipment, this tremendous gift God has giving us called the human body, the child has been taken out of action, the child has been taken out of commission, the child has been put on lockdown!

Can you imagine the confusion and trauma that this child is facing now? The child was feeling so happy moving around and receiving our approval and acceptance for getting and giving us something and now for that very act they are being punished. And OHYEAH American, the child knows it is being punished, how can we tell?

Did you ever notice how when we put our children in one of those "Child Prisons", how they respond to being captured? They start screaming and kicking and hollering and making all kinds of protests because they know that they should be out running and not cooped up in a little **"Kiddie Prison"** sometimes for hours at a time.

The child knows that the joy it had received from moving around, from walking around, from playing around has now been taking from it and it is MAD!

BUT CAN YOU BLAME IT AMERICA!

Let us tell you about one more part of our Theory America that seems to happen quite a bit in our country. Because we are a very busy society, or at least had been until this recent downturn, we seem to find other ways to deal with our responsibility of taking care of our children. We are not criticizing anyone we are just noting a trend in our society in the last 40 years or so. Most of the time in most households both parents are working. Because of this, there was an extreme proliferation of children being cared for away from the home.

Now we are not downing day cares or working mothers so please do not look upon these statements we are going to make as being such. But we want to make it very clear that we believe that no one, no one is ever going to be any better nurturer for their child then a loving, caring and concerned mother! That kind of mother does not look upon her role in motherhood as a job but as her calling for life.

Just let me say America and I know you have heard it often: **There Ain't No Love Like a Mother's Love!** Mothers will do without for their children!

Mothers will do without food, clothing, shoes and whatever else they have to for their children. Mother's will die for their children. When mothers had the luxury and the ability to be able to stay at home they were able to make sure that every aspect of the child's life was in proper order and the mother gave the child the best she had!

And because mothers had the opportunity of being with that child all day long the mother could make whatever adjustments in the child's
 life the child needed help in, a good diet, a good education and a good physical fitness program that would promote the child's health to the best of her ability.And there was urgency for the mother to do whatever she could to help this child obtain whatever it needed for it to have the best that she could give it.

And we knew that when mother told us that we were overweight or needed to lose a couple of pounds she was not doing it to degrade us or to make fun of us, Butt she was doing it to help us. And those stay-at-home mothers knew just what to do to get us to do what it was that they wanted us to do. Sometimes it might be with honey and sometimes it might have been with vinegar, *"Butt she got her done!"*

It was never a case of whose responsibility it was to take care of every aspect of her child's life. It was clear in her mind that this child was her responsibility and that every aspect of its care was her responsibility.

Chapter 8    Who's Responsible Now!

We are not downing you for putting your children in day care because that's not the point we are making. But because of our fast-paced lives it is easy for us not to have the time necessary to spend with our children and make sure that they are getting the right amount of physical fitness that they need or the proper type that is required to provide them with overall good fitness & good health.

We normally think they will get it in the day care, or when they get older in the schools but there is a unique relationship between the home, the day care and later the school which must be explored and addressed.

In a recent article on the Center For Disease Control website titled Community Activity Programs Are Money in the Bank it showed the unique relationship between the home and any other entity such as schools, day cares, social support networks were very beneficial in helping whole communities to become physically fit. It is very important for us all to consider this article and its implications.

Because one of the greatest parts of the article is that we all need to be looking for a way to resolve this problems plaguing our communities. In a related article on Yahoo health titled Childhood Obesity, when asked why are so many children obese Dr. David Ludwig MD, Phd said that genetic factors sometimes play a role in a child's being overweight however in the past 30 years genetics has not changed. The recent tripling in the obesity rate can therefore only be attributed to the environmental factors.

He went on to say that two thirds of our obesity problem would vanish if we revert back to the way we did things 40 years ago. We need to stop consuming so many fast foods, soft drinks and a high glycemic index foods. He said parent's efforts to teach their children how to eat healthy foods are being undermined by advertisements on TV.

Children who spend several hours watching television have not developed any athletic skills or love of physical fitness that can make athletics and staying fit for a lifetime more fun and enjoyable as they grow into adults. Dr. Ludwig goes on to say everyone is working too hard and too long and that we are not spending enough time with our children to teach them about good nutrition and the benefits of being physically active and or being physically active with them.

40 years ago families cooked dinner and sat down and ate together on a regular basis. Too often now dinner is picked up at a fast food restaurant and eaten on the go. There is no alternative to a parent cooking a dinner and setting down with his or her children and eating together and then going outside to play. The answer to the obesity epidemic is very simple Dr. Ludwig says. We need to get back to more traditional ways of eating, exercising and being with family.

As we said when we began this chapter Who's Responsible Now! We do not want to put the blame on or criticize any one group because from all of the related articles we are seeing that to blame anyone it would be an indictment of everyone, America. Because it's our American lifestyle and our pursuit of all of these materialistic things that have gotten in the way of what is really important, and what really has value, which is our families, America, our people, US.

And just as we have gotten into this situation we can get ourselves out of this situation, But it is not going to be easy, and is going to require some work, BUTT we can do it America.
Because America, we Americans have never looked for the easy way out and we've always been able to work hard.  This is a battle that we cannot afford to lose.  This is a battle that we have got to win.  This is a battle that if we do not win then we will  DY-

BUTT

We Are Not Going To Let You

DY-BUTT LIVE!
DO
DYBUTT & LIVE!

Chapter 9   What is Dynamic Muscular Breakthrough Technology!
(DYBUTT)

America, it is with great pleasure that we introduce you to, DRUM ROLL PLEASE Dynamic Muscular Breakthrough Technology! Once in awhile a product comes along that is just perfect for the times. That is what Dynamic Muscular Breakthrough Technology is! It is a breakthrough in fitness technology BUTT it is also our philosophy as well. Let's take a look at the fitness part first shall we?

Dynamic= the effects of forces on the motion of an object. The word has a Greek origin whose etymology is from the ancient Greek dynamis meaning strength or power. The definition is from the branch of mechanics that is concerned with the effects of forces on the motion of objects. This definition was used because we want you to become the powerful mechanical entity known as the DYBUTT Machine!

Muscular= the ability to produce force and to cause motion in the body's contactile tissue in the physiological sense, may involve shortening and changing shape, or it may generate force without any change in length.

As the DYBUTT machine you will learn to generate force and cause motion in such a way as to enhance your cardiovascular and muscular fitness.

Breakthrough= a sudden rush to the solution of a problem. Our problem as a nation is that we are faced with An Obesity Epidemic as never before. Butt we have the solution to that problem and it is DYBUTT.

Technology= The means, the methods, technique & the knowledge man uses to control his environment. DYBUTT is going to change the way the world works out. You will learn how to control your physical environment by using DYBUTT!

Dybutt is the physical fitness component that every individual needs. It not only provides a cardiovascular and a muscle building /toning component at the same time. It does it without the use of any weights, belts, bands, pulleys, machines or equipment of any kind. It's based upon the principles of isometrics, isokinetics and isotonics. Now why were these principles important? They allow for the development of muscle strength, power, endurance, stamina, stability, shape and definition. And one's own body could be used as the resistances thus eliminating the need for any special equipment or apparatuses.

We will put a definition of the terms here

**ISOMETRIC EXERCISE.** During isometric exercises muscles contract; however, there is no motion in the affected joints. The muscle fibers maintain a constant length throughout the entire contraction. Isometric training is effective for developing total strength of a particular muscle or group of muscles. It is often used for rehabilitation, since the exact area of muscle weakness can be isolated and strengthening can be administered at the proper joint angle. This kind of training can provide a relatively quick and convenient method for overloading and strengthening muscles without any special equipment and with little chance of injury.

**ISOKINETIC EXERCISE.** Isokinetic exercise controls the speed of movement within the range of motion. Isokinetic exercise attempts to combine the best features of both isometrics and we ight training. It is resistive exercise utilizing a fixed speed and variable resistance. It provides muscular overload at a constant preset speed while the muscle mobilizes its force through the full range of motion.

**ISOTONIC EXERCISE.** Isotonic exercise differs from isometric exercise in that there is movement of the joint during the **muscle contraction**. It is exercise with a fixed resistance and variable speed. A classic example of an isotonic exercise is weight training with dumbbells and barbells. As the weight is lifted throughout the range of motion, the muscle shortens and lengthens.

The DYBUTT dance program also uses the trademarked Maximum Major Muscle Engagement techniques that encourages the engagement of as many of the bodies major muscles groups as is possible. This causes a synergistic effect that permits a great cardiovascular and muscle-toning workout in about 10 to 20 minutes! The varying intensity of the Interval Training principle is also used to provide an even better fitness experience.

There is also new research that shows that the multitasking movements used in Dybutt could develop more neurons & neurons brain pathways, which could cause its participants to become smarter!

With the DYBUTT Dance Fitness Program you are in total control of the amount of pressure and exertion you use to perform your movements. You can use a light, moderate or high level of intense pressure to challenge the muscles of your body to optimum effort resulting in maximum strength, growth, toning & cardio development by eliminating the need to do endless repetitions and going right to the point of Maximum Major Muscle Engagement immediately.

We hope that these definitions have provided some clarity for you on why this is the greatest workout program and the last program you will

84

ever need! It will provide you with a fantastic workout in any environment that you want to use because the only piece of equipment you need is you. We have a quote from our website that we would like to share with you about our product:

This is the most unique, new, efficient, scientific and easy workout program that you will ever experience. With DYBUTT you'll be able to get a full Total Body resistance and cardiovascular workout in about 20 minutes. Without the use of weights, machines, bands, pulleys or any other special equipment.

There is no jumping or heavy lifting of weights involved in the dance. There is no hanging from bars or doing chin-ups or pull-ups or push-ups involved in the program. And the program features an abdominal development component that can be done without ever getting on the floor again. It is designed to put as little stress, wear and tear on the joints, ligaments and tendons as is possible.

Truly this is the fitness program for the 25th century that is available today and there are several ways to participate listed below:
we can participate individually by using DVDs, in class form by either DVD or by personal instruction. There are now eight DVDs that are available and each one of them is designed to provide you with the optimum in physical fitness and health.

Our DVDs and fitness programs run in length

from our fitness express program that is only 20 minutes long and provides a great total body cardio/muscle-toning/building workout in 20 minutes. To our 45 minutes Dynamic Muscular Breakthrough Technology, DYBUTT for Hard Times DVD that uses water bottles and cans as resistance. And oh yeah we do have one DVD that does use weights and it is a tremendous workout! Only Mark can do it so far!

Dynamic Muscular Breakthrough Technology is also a multi-generational fitness program and what's so good about that you asked?
The great thing is that the same things that children are learning in school or day care are the same things that you can do at home. Or the family can work out with them when they come home. One of our students is three years old and our oldest student is eighty-three years of age.

This is a program that we can use for the rest of our lives! And because Dybutt is so fluid and user-friendly one can use many different kinds of movement and many different kinds of music to perform our fitness program. We are not chained down to just one type of workout or one type of music but we can use multiple types of movements and music to perform our DYBUTT physical fitness program.

The Center For Disease Control, (CDC) reports that everyone no matter what age group we are in, needs to have a physical fitness program that provides a cardiovascular and a muscle toning/building component. For elementary school youth they need to have at least ½ to an hour per day of moderate to vigorous physical activity, with two sessions to include muscle toning/building movements or exercises.

Middle school and high school students need at least 45 minutes of moderate to vigorous activity per day, with at least two sessions to include muscle toning/building movements or exercises.

It was also noted that adults need 30 minutes per day of cardiovascular activity and two sessions per week of muscle toning/building exercises to have the right amount of physical fitness for a well-rounded physical fitness program. Dynamic Muscular Breakthrough Technology or DYBUTT, provides and exceeds those requirements necessary for us to have the kind of fitness program that will provide us with great health and physical fitness.

But DYBUTT provides us with a bonus that other programs don't.

DYBUTT does all of this without the use of any weights, bands, belts, pulleys, machines, apparatuses, or equipment of any kind and we can do it anywhere at anytime without the need at any special facilities. That means all we have to do is take the time to do DYBUTT, and besides for the cost of the DVD, that's the extent of the investment that we will have to make to have a fitness program that will meet all of our fitness needs and goals for the rest of our lives!

But that's not the only extra bonus that Dybutt provides! Because we did not have to purchase or use any extra equipment there is nothing to set up, cleanup, disinfect, put away or store. When we decide to have a DYBUTT fitness class all we really need is a place to perform the movements in. And that could be an existing room such as a bathroom, bedroom, living room, kitchen, basement, classroom, conference room, meeting room, church meeting hall, backyard, deck, or any other place that we can take our DVD player or our computer!

I know you're going to find it hard to believe America, but there's still more benefits associated with the Dynamic Muscular Breakthrough Technology or DYBUTT fitness program! As certified personal trainers, we have noticed that one of the most prevalent complaints that people have about becoming involved in a physical fitness program is the fact that many of the exercises are just too difficult for them to perform.

We personally believe that that is a reason why 2/3rds of all Americans do not exercise and about 2/3rds of all Americans are overweight.

And a lot of people come to the conclusion that we Americans are overweight because we are lazy. **But We Do Not Believe That! We believe that the reason why two thirds of Americans do not exercise is not because they're lazy; it is because the exercise experience and fitness programs to this point have been so**

# **CRAAZZZY!!**

**Because so many of the exercises put so much stress & cause so much damage to our joints, ligaments, tendons, cartilage & other connective & soft tissue that exercise has**

<u>become a very painful and unpleasant</u>
<u>experience!</u> **WE DO NOT BELIEVE IN THE NO PAIN NO GAIN FORM OF PHYSICAL FITNESS!**

## WE BELIEVE THAT "NO PAIN NO GAIN IS NO GOOD!!"

That is one of the major advantages of DYBUTT; it is soo easy on our joint, ligaments, tendons, cartilage, and other connective tissues! What does that mean America; it means that now we have a workout program that we can do without doing damage to those areas!

If we're not hurting America maybe we will be willing to participate in a physical education program. Maybe that two thirds, after being made aware of the fact that they need to exercise at least 30 minutes per day and that 2 of those sessions need to be muscle toning/building sessions, in order for them not to DY-BUTT LIVE they will began to do our DYBUTT fitness program and LIVE!

90

And you know what America, The Center for Disease Control, (CDC) is reporting that as long as we get at least 10 minutes of moderate to vigorous exercise that that will count towards our 30 minute total for the day.  Isn't that great news! Because what that means is that we can get 10 minutes in the morning, 10 minutes aft er lunchtime and 10 minutes after dinner time and we have our 30 minute total in for the day.  What a great way to get into fantastic physical condition doing it 10 minutes at a time three times a day any and everywhere that you decide to do it without any special equipment.  JUST YOU!

**YOU**

# BECOME THE DYBUTT MACHINE!!!

Chapter 10 The Dynamic Muscular Breakthrough Technology

(DYBUTT) PHILOSOPHY!

Kathy and I believe in a very simple philosophy and it is this America. All of our lives we are going to have challenges, sometimes for all our lives we will be challenged. No matter who we are this is a fact. Rich people are challenged, middle-class people are challenged, poor people are challenged. Smart people, & not so smart people, workers and employers, young people & I don't like to use the word old but vintaged, vintage people are challenged. Everyone!

# BUTT we must decide how we will handle those challenges!

**We can decide to let these challenges stop us or**

we can decide that in spite of the challenges we are going to succeed!  We must start looking at challenges not as points that are going to prevent us from achieving what it is we should achieve, BUTT we must start to look at every challenge as an opportunity for great glory and success! We must think that the harder and bigger the challenge maybe, the greater our victory will be when we overcome it America! No one would think it was a great big deal or such a great accomplishment if we were to go out and beat Judge Judy in a game of one-on-one, so what!  But now if we were to go out and beat Lebron James in a game of one on one now that would be something!

We have a big challenge before us

America, the CDC is reporting that 1000 of us Americans are going to die today from obesity related or fat diseases!  They are predicting that this is going to be the first generation that will have a shorter life expectancy then their parents. BUTT the CDC made an additional statement and it was this America.  They said with intervention these deaths could be avoided!  In other words, if we can do something that will help us to start eating right and starts exercising right then we can stop all this DYING!  America, Dynamic Muscular Breakthrough Technology (DYBUTT) is the intervention that is going to stop all this DYING!

BUTT America we have to start doing the program!  And we know America that it is very easy to make many different excuses for not doing the program. And we hear those excuses, excuses such as these: I would work out BUTT I just don't have the time. With our programs we can do them in 10 minutes increments and get a fantastic cardiovascular and muscle toning/building workout at the same time. I would work out BUTT I don't know what to do. We show you in very easy to understand language and movements what to do.

We have a student as young as three years old that can do most of the movements. I would work out BUTT those high impact movements hurt my feet, ankles, knees and hips. With most our programs your feet never leave the floor thus preventing any high impact aerobic injuries. We do have some for our more advanced students and athletes that do have some impact to them. I would work out BUTT I hate lifting weights. With most of our programs you don't have to use any kind of equipment including weights. You learn movements that will allow you to become the only piece of machinery that you need!

You become the DYBUTT MACHINE!

One of the favorite that we hear America, is I would work out but I'm just too old and I hurt so badly. DYBUTT is so user and joint friendly, that it is the perfect workout for those who are advanced in years. We presently have a student that is 83 years old and he thinks the program is great. What DYBUTT does is make the areas of the body that tend to become old and feeble strong and flexible. And it does its in a very safe, controllable and effective manner.

We believe that there is a BUTT that gets in the way of many successes. I would've been a great student, BUTT I didn't like to study. I would've been a great athlete, BUTT I didn't like to practice. I wouldn't have hit him, BUTT I couldn't control myself.

DYBUTT takes every excuse that we may have for not being fit, looking great, and being in great health and not dying and DYBUTT kills it, eliminates it, destroys its, or makes it DY.

America, they said a thousand of us are going to die today BUTT we at DYBUTT say we are not going to DY-BUTT LIVE! They say that this will be the first generation

97

whose children will die before them.  But we at DYBUTT believe that The Children are not going to DY-BUTT LIVE!  America, we shall not DY-BUTT LIVE because we have the intervention that will prevent the thousand from DYING today!  We have the intervention that will prevent The Children from DYING before their parents!

America, we must start doing DYBUTT NOW, TODAY so that's we can reverse this trend and stop DYING and start living NOW! JOIN THE DYBUTT CAMPAIGN NOW! GO TO www.dybutt.com & buy a DVD for our children, our parents, our schools, for us & let's start to beat this obesity epidemic NOW! America, we know that it is going to be challenging for us to get back to the level of physical fitness and health that we enjoyed 40 years ago! Please note, we do not blame any one single group, not mothers, not fathers, not daycares, not schools, or even individuals. Because blaming anyone would be an indictment for everyone. So placing the blame really is useless because we are where we are as a nation. But America, we must & we shall solve this problem as a nation!

As the Psalmists wrote in Psalm 118: 17;

# "I SHALL NOT DIE, BUT LIVE AND DECLARE THE WORKS OF THE LORD"

**MAY GOD BLESS AMERICA &**

**MAY GOD BLESS YOU!**

**LOVE YOU, Rev. Dr. MARK D. &**

**KATHY M. BROWN, I.**

**Stop Dying & Start Living ,America!**

**Do Dybutt!**

www.ingramcontent.com/pod-product-compliance
Lightning Source LLC
Chambersburg PA
CBHW060637290526
45793CB00001B/286